Busy Fami
Can Eat Clean...

Tips to Make Clean Eating a Part of your Family's Life

Dottie Copps

CKβ Publishing

ISBN-13:

9780692231975 (CKB Publishing)

ISBN-10:

069231978

Introduction

Today, busy seems to be the common word that defines any family. Whether you have multiple children and you find yourself running to activity after activity or you are a two person family with many obligations, time can easily get away from you. Unfortunately, the one place that seems to suffer the most when we become busy is our meals. We tend to turn to unhealthy food just to save time. Whether it is because you believe that healthy food takes too long to prepare, it costs too much money or you just do not know where to start – there are simple ways to incorporate healthy, clean eating meals into your family's routine.

Eating healthy does not take hours of preparation; it probably even takes less time than it might take to go to a fast food restaurant or to cook a frozen meal. The food industry has led us all to believe that convenience food is the way to go because it gets you out the door in a flash or it helps busy parents have dinner on the table moments after walking in the door. To make matters worse, the food industry has even made us believe that some of this food is "healthy." Unfortunately, the exact opposite is true – no matter how low fat or reduced sugar an item is, there are additives making up for the lack in taste to make consumers come back for more.

According to the Robert Wood Johnson Foundation, there are thirteen states that have obesity rates over 30 percent and 41 states that have above a 25 percent obesity rate. To make matters worse, no state fell below the 20 percent obesity rate in the study. Of course, these statistics vary by region, age and gender, but the overall idea is that these rates are too high. Everyone has their own reason for the amount that they weigh and no two people that are obese have the same reason. This also means that there is not a cut and dry solution to help those that are overweight. Even those people that are not overweight are at risk for serious, chronic and life threatening diseases if they do not eat right. The common denominator in all of this is understanding what you eat and how it affects your body.

Clean eating can help a variety of issues including assisting in losing weight, fighting chronic disease, fighting mental illness and having an overall feeling of wellbeing. Clean eating does not mean that you will never eat another hamburger again or that you have to live on salad and water for the rest of your life. It also does not mean that you will spend hours in the kitchen, slaving over food that does not even taste good. It means a simple change in your lifestyle, the way that you look at food and what you choose to eat.

Yes, in the beginning it might be challenging to get started just because it will be a different way of life. It will take a little more preparation, but this book will help you learn how to handle it to allow for the least amount of work and time. Your body has likely been trained to look for food that you think tastes good, but it is simply a mask for the genuine natural food that your body should be enjoying. After reading this book, you will learn how to adjust your mind, body and taste buds to enjoy the natural foods in life.

This book will also help you learn how to get your entire family on board with your new clean eating routine. You will learn how to read labels, understand what sugar and refined foods are doing to your body and how to ditch those habits and incorporate a clean eating lifestyle. It is not as hard as it sounds and before long you will wonder how you ever ate any other way.

Chapter 1 – Define your Family's Rules

When your family is stuck on their habits, introducing a new way of life or even a new food once in a while can be extremely difficult. This might make changing overall habits seem downright impossible, especially if you have finicky children – but it is possible! Before you do anything, it is best to sit down and talk through your plans with everyone. You can start by discussing the positives of this new clean eating lifestyle. When you show your children how much they can benefit by choosing these new habits, they might be more willing to jump on board. A few of the positives that you can offer include:

- **Everyone will be healthier** - If your kids despise the common cold or the stomach flu as much as the rest of us, this should be incentive enough. When clean, healthy foods are chosen, the immune system naturally becomes stronger making illnesses and gross tasting medicines a thing of the past.

- **Mom and dad will have more energy** - If you are like most parents, you are run down and exhausted by the end of the day. But guess who is not tired? That's right the kids continue to run circles around us as we would give anything for five minutes of rest. When you change to a clean eating diet, however, your energy will naturally increase because your body does not have to waste energy on digesting chemicals, additives and preservatives. This means that you will have more energy to be with your kids.

- **Stomachaches will go away** – If you have children that get chronic upset stomachs or suffer from constipation, they will love how they feel on a clean eating diet. They will begin having regular bowel movements and will spend less time laying down missing out on activities because their stomach hurts.

- **Skin outbreaks will decrease** – If you have any teenagers in your life, they will love this reason! Sugar and toxins play a large role in how a teen's skin appears. Acne, dry skin and other skin blemishes can be a result of a poor diet. Encourage your teen to try this new diet, if only for a while, to see how their skin reacts. Soon enough, you will not have to say anything; the food will speak for itself.

These are just a few of the reasons that might pertain to kids or at the very least, give them the desire to try it out with you. If there is illness that runs in your family, you can talk about how choosing the right foods can help to keep those illnesses away from you and your children. These talks will obviously depend on the age of your children and the level of what they can understand. The most important factor here is that everyone is involved in the decision making process to ensure that the new lifestyle is accepted by everyone.

What Are The Rules?

Every household will have their own clean eating rules. You do not even have to call them rules, because as we all know, some kids will rebel just hearing the word rules! Come up with your own word that you know your children will not rebel against and will instead accept and even be excited about. Below are some guidelines on what your rules could look like:

- Eat only whole foods, including whole grains

- Reduce the consumption of refined sugar (including artificial sweeteners)

- Try to avoid fast food

- Eat very little food from a box (learn to read ingredients)

- Only drink real drinks – nothing processed
- Eat as many whole fruits and vegetables as desired

- Eat organic dairy

- Use natural sweeteners sparingly

- Consume only homemade meals and snacks rather than prepackaged choices

Your family's rules could look similar to these or completely different. It is up to you and your family on how you incorporate this new eating plan into your lifestyle. When you are making your rules, try to avoid using words like "Don't, Avoid and Off Limits." Those words for kids are like an invitation to break the rules. Instead, you want to make this change a positive change for everyone. You do not want your children or the adults in your family to feel deprived – you want them to feel empowered. They should come out of the family meeting thinking that they can do this and that they will feel great – not begrudging this next move and hoping that it is a phase that does not last long.

If some of your family members get upset at the new "rules", try to put a positive spin on them. Instead of saying "don't eat those cookies for a snack," try something like, "let's try a new snack today" and introduce a new homemade clean eating fruit dip served with a favorite fruit. Yes, this snack might not look as pleasing to someone's trained eye that has learned to eat cookies after school, but once the fruit dip and fruit are given a chance, they will become a treat too.

Make Small Changes

Once your family has defined the rules that everyone can live with, it is time to start making changes. Before you jump in head first, it is important to determine how you want to make those changes. If you have young kids, it is easier to take baby steps. For busy families, small changes are typically best because they allow everyone to adapt and they do not take a lot of your time or effort to implement. You should start by choosing one area to change at a time to see how your family reacts. Following are some of the changes you will need to make in the end – you can decide what works/doesn't work for your family and make your individual plan and starting point from there.

Add New Foods Slowly

When you add new foods slowly, you give everyone a chance to get acclimated to them one at a time. This means adding a new fruit, vegetable or whole grain to your diet weekly in the beginning. You can advance to daily once everyone becomes more accepting of the new diet. This slow method gives everyone a chance to determine what they do and do not like. Changes such as switching from white bread to whole grain bread could be very difficult, especially for kids, so it is important to take your time.

Research has shown that it takes up to 10 tries before anyone can decide if they like a new food. This means do not give up! If everyone resists the way that you served a new fruit, vegetable or whole grain the first time, try it a different way the next time to see if you get a more positive response.

In the case of white bread, encourage everyone to just keep trying. If they are truly resistant, you can ditch the bread all together and provide alternative healthy lunches for your children or even yourself until your taste buds are ready to accept the delicious whole grain versions. The most important thing to remember is not to give up. This lifestyle change takes time as everyone's taste buds need to slowly come back to enjoying the basic foods rather than the processed tastes that we have all become accustomed to.

Change Your Drinks

The one drink that is perfectly acceptable on a clean eating diet is water, but not everyone wants to live on water alone, especially kids! Luckily there are simple ways to incorporate healthy drinks and eliminate soda, sweetened juice and sugar filled coffee. For adults, coffee and tea are acceptable, it is the sugar and additive filled creamers that are not. It is easiest if you slowly wean yourself off of those habits rather than drastically pulling them from your diet. You can still drink your coffee, which means you will still get caffeine, it just will not be as sweet as you are used to drinking, which might take a little time. If your kids are hooked on juice, try to purchase only natural juice. This means that the juice should not be from concentrate and the only ingredients should be those that the juice is made from. For example, orange juice should only have oranges or carrot juice should only have carrots as their ingredients.

Pack Healthy Lunches

If you pack lunch for you or your kids, it is about to change. Think about what you pack right now. Does your lunch sack include a lot of prepackaged goodies? On a clean eating diet, those are not considered goodies. Instead, you will pack real, wholesome food that will fuel the body throughout the day rather than drag it down. Packing healthy lunches will not take much longer than it takes you to pack your lunch now. You have simply been trained to rely on convenience foods because they are "fast", but you will soon learn how fast healthy lunches can be too.

Snack Healthy

Snacks are a difficult area to change because they are typically the grab-and-go type foods. It might take a little planning in this area, but once you get started, it is easy to maintain healthy snacks. Rather than going to the pantry and grabbing chips or crackers, try going to the refrigerator and grabbing whole fruit, vegetables or low-fat/organic dairy. The easiest way to make healthy snacking successful is to prepackage all of the snacks at the beginning of the week. Then you get that same grab-and-go feeling without the unnecessary additives and preservatives.

Use Fewer Ingredients

One of the most amazing things about the clean eating diet is the decreased amount of ingredients that you need to use when you prepare snacks and meals. When you eat foods in as close to the whole form as possible, you do not need to add refined sugars, flours and other additives. The foods taste great on their own.

As you navigate your way on this diet, you will see how simple it is to recreate the recipes simply because of the very few ingredients that you need. Not only will this enhance your health, but it will save you numerous trips to the grocery store, which all busy families know, is a highly sought after goal!

As we move through the chapters in this book, you will walk through each step of a clean eating diet to help everyone in your family slowly adapt to this new way of life. You will learn why you should choose whole grains rather than refined grains or why sugar is so bad for you. You will also learn how to read labels to see what you are eating and how to put it all together. In the long run, you will love the way that you feel and will hopefully never go back to choosing processed foods. You have made the first step in achieving a healthy family, regardless of how busy you are; now it is time to continue the journey and help enhance the health of those that you love most.

Chapter 2 – Why Low Fat Or Low Sugar Foods Are Not As Healthy As You Think

When you are at the store, do you gravitate towards foods that are labeled low-fat or low sugar? The good news is that you are not alone, many people do that too. The bad news is that just as you should not judge a book by its cover; you should not judge food by its packaging. Low fat, low sugar, high fiber or even the word healthy are all words that the food manufacturers have adopted in the face of the public becoming much more health conscious. What they rely on is the fact that most people do not read nutrition labels or even if they do, they do not know what they are reading. It is time to put a stop to that because you are not doing yourself or your family any good. In fact, you could be harming your body with ingredients that you did not even realize that you were consuming.

Learning the Truth

First, we need to learn what the various terms that food labels can carry mean, according to the FDA and the USDA.

- Foods that contain 0.5 grams of fat or less per serving are considered fat free

- Foods that contain less than or equal to 3 grams of fat per serving are considered low fat

- Foods that have a reduced fat content of 25 percent off of the original can be considered reduced fat

- Foods that have half of the fat content or 33 percent fewer calories than the original can be considered light

The problem with the labeling is that you cannot rely on fat or calorie content alone. If these foods were left on their own, with no ingredients added, the fat-free and low-fat versions would not taste good. In fact, most people likely would not eat them. So what does the food industry do?

They add ingredients into the food that does not alter the fat content, but might alter the calories, not to mention making them unhealthy because the ingredients typically include sugar, an artificial sweetener, salt or other harmful additives that we cannot even pronounce.

It does not matter what is on the label of a particular food; if it is processed in any way, it is not good for you.

Processed foods are altered in a way that takes the food far away from its natural state, removing its nutrients and replacing them with harmful chemicals. Unfortunately, we are trained to think that only fattening foods are processed and bad for you, when the truth is there are numerous low-fat or non-fat foods that are just as bad, if not worse for you.

Saturated Fat

The problem that most of us have fallen prey to is avoiding saturated fat, which has been named the "bad guy" when it comes to food. We are all aware of it and it is what started the low-fat craze. Food manufacturers began removing saturated fat, but to retain the good taste of these foods, began replacing them with refined sugar and carbs, which translates into many more calories. So consumers that think that they are choosing "healthy" food because they are low in fat could be consuming more calories than the original product. It is a deceiving process that the food industry has capitalized on and is what has caused waistlines to expand and diseases to skyrocket.

Good Fat vs Bad Fat

You have likely heard the term "good fat" before. It is true, there are good fats that your body needs to survive. These good fats are monounsaturated and polyunsaturated fats. The bad fats are saturated and trans fat. The good fats are found in whole, healthy foods including vegetable oil, nuts and Omega-3 rich fish.

They are not found in processed, low-fat foods. The best way to think about it is to consume foods that contain good fat, not those that are non-fat. This is especially important for children. The right fat intake is essential for a child's brain and nervous system to properly develop. Let's take a closer look at the different types of fats:

- Unsaturated Fats – There are three types of unsaturated fats; monounsaturated, polyunsaturated and Omega-3 fatty acids. These fats are considered neutral, meaning they do no harm and actually help the body.

- Saturated Fats – These are the bad fats. They are found in processed baked goods as well as meat and full fat dairy.

- Trans Fats – These are also bad fats. They are found in processed foods, butter and fried foods. They are also called partially hydrogenated oils on some labels.

The American Heart Association recommends that children between the ages of 2 and 3 consume between 30 and 35 percent of their calories in the form of good fat and children ages 4 to 18 get between 25 and 35 percent of their calories from good fat. It is important to know that one fat gram equals 9 calories, which could help you figure out how many grams of fat your child should be consuming.

 For example, an average 4-8 year old female should consume an average of 1,200 calories. This means that she should consume around 40 grams of good fat per day. This fat is good fat though, which means vegetable oils, nuts, avocados and Omega-3 rich foods.

Any saturated fat consumption should be limited to 10 percent of any child's diet, regardless of age. In a standard 1,300 calorie diet, this equals only 14 grams of fat, which if you looked at the labels of some of the cookies, cakes, chips or other foods that children eat, it does not take much to reach that level. Of course, these levels depend on your child's health and level of activity and should be discussed with his/her doctor.

A Prime Example

Let's take a look at the difference between the consumption of low-fat salad dressing and wholesome, dressing that contains a little fat to get an idea of how low-fat foods are ruining us. Salad dressing is an area that many people tend to opt for the low-fat version, thinking that they are doing their body good by cutting calories. A study done by Purdue University helps us to see why choosing the low-fat version is not doing our bodies any good.

In this study, participants were each given salad filled with a variety of vegetables. Each participant was then given different types of dressings; a monounsaturated dressing (canola oil), polyunsaturated fat dressing (soybean oil) and saturated fat dressing (butter). After consumption, each participant had their blood tested to see how well the nutrients in the vegetables, including lutein, lycopene and beta-carotene were absorbed.

The study found that those that consumed the monounsaturated fat dressing, which can be found in canola or olive oil dressings, had the greatest results. This means that when you choose low-fat or fat-free dressings, you are negating the value of eating a nutrient rich salad because your body is not absorbing the fat soluble vitamins. In addition, you could be consuming larger amounts of calories and sugar – doing your body even more harm.

The Truth About Low Sugar Foods

If think that you are doing your body good by consuming low-sugar foods, you might be in for a surprise. Let's take a look, for example, at diet soda. A quick glance at a can will show you that there are zero grams of sugar in it. Does that make it healthy? The answer is obviously, no. Diet soda or any other food/drink that is labeled "low sugar" could do your body more harm than the foods that contain the sugar.

This is because of what is used to replace the sugar – artificial sweeteners. The food or drink needs to get its sweet taste from somewhere and artificial sweeteners are even sweeter than regular sugar. There is a huge problem with these sweeteners; they mess with your brain, resulting in damage to your body. Let's take a look:

When you consume a food that contains artificial sweetener, you are playing tricks on your body. When your taste buds get a hold of the sweet taste of the product made with artificial sweetener, (which is extremely sweet because artificial sweeteners are much sweeter than sugar) your brain gets ready to produce dopamine, as it would with sugar consumption.

The only problem is that there is no sugar hitting the brain, which leaves your brain confused and craving more sweets. This could cause you to reach for even more sugary foods or eat too many calories to make up for the void that the artificial sweetener has left behind.

As we go through this book, you will learn how to recognize the ingredients in foods, learning how to decipher the various names for artificial sweeteners so that you can avoid them in your diet.

High Fiber – Is It A Hoax?

Today, many food labels scream the words "HIGH FIBER" at you. They want to grab your attention and let you know that these foods are high in fiber. While this might be true; what it does not say is that these products are also high in sugar, fat and calories. Any processed cake, cookie or cereal that suddenly has "added fiber" needs to make up for that taste somewhere else. The best way that food manufacturers know to do that is with added sugar and fat.

Rather than turning to these so-called high fiber foods, the best place to get fiber for you and your family is through whole fruits and vegetables. This will give you the highest amount of fiber as well as the other vital vitamins and nutrients that a varied diet provides.

Lesson Learned

Now that you know that low-fat, low sugar and high in fiber are simply ways to reel you in to buy products that are not nearly as good for you as the real thing, you can start to adapt your family's diet to one that is cleaner and healthier. It will take some planning and a bit of patience, but with time and plenty of recipes, you will be able to replicate the foods that your family has learned to love, just in a much healthier way.

Homework

Before you move on to the next chapter, take a moment to go through your pantry. Take inventory of every processed food item that you have. Take a close look at the sugar and fat content. We will discuss the other ingredients in future chapters. At this point, your homework is to simply choose one thing from a shelf to toss. It can be low-fat, full fat or loaded with artificial sweeteners. L

et everyone in your family agree on the item that will no longer enter your home. If everyone is ready, try to let each family member choose one thing, then you can rid your home of even more unhealthy food and make room for the good, clean food that you are about to discover.

Chapter 3 - Learning to Read Ingredient Labels

Have you realized the traps that you have fallen into when it comes to processed foods yet? Those foods that so innocently claim to be healthy, whether they say "now contains more fiber" or "low fat," "low calorie" or "fortified with vitamins," are not healthy. They are still processed foods that might contain a few "good things" added back into them – but they are nowhere near as good as the real thing. Take the time to look at the ingredient list, even if you are not sure what you are looking at just yet, if there are more than a handful of ingredients, the product is not good for you. These products that contain 20 or more ingredients than necessary, including high amounts of salt and sugar, are only providing your family with empty calories.

Know Your Ingredients

The best weapon that you have against eating processed foods is reading the ingredients. As a general rule, foods that contain more than five ingredients are processed to some degree. This does not mean that all foods that have more than five ingredients are bad for you, but careful attention should be paid. To make matters worse – most of these products that contain chemicals, sweeteners, artificial flavors and other additives created in a factory also have the good, nutrient-rich ingredients stripped from them. This leaves you with food that does not do anything good for your body.

As a general rule, if you do not know an ingredient or cannot pronounce it, then you should not be eating it. As you go down the list, ask yourself if you would use those ingredients in recipes that you make at home. If the answer is "no" then you should not be eating them in processed foods. Let's take a look at a few of the most popular ingredients that you want to steer clear of:

- **BHA** – This ingredient, which can be found on ingredient lists as butylated hydroxyanisole, has mixed reviews. It is approved by the FDA in small amounts, but researchers have found that it causes cancer in the forestomachs of rats. Because humans do not have a forestomach, it is considered relatively safe. But do you want to take that chance? This ingredient is most commonly found in the following foods: potato chips, instant mashed potatoes, some cereals, gum, baked goods and preserved meat (lunch meat). It is also found in many household products! Its main purpose is to prevent the fat in the product from becoming rancid when it hits the air.

- **Partially Hydrogenated Oil** – This ingredient has been touched upon already, but it is important to know its danger. The FDA has deemed it permissible for food manufacturers to claim that a food has 0 grams of trans-fat as long as it has less than .5 grams per serving. This means that your food can contain as much as .49 grams of trans fat per serving and still be labeled "no trans-fat." It is vital that you look for this ingredient in the ingredient list, rather than relying on the claims on the front of the package. Case in point, if you were to consume 5 items that contained .49 grams of trans fat, you would be over the 2 grams of trans fat per day that is considered the maximum amount to be consumed in order to avoid serious cardiovascular issues. This is very easy to do considering trans-fat is found in muffins, cakes, pastas, cereals and microwave popcorn, just to name a few items.

- **Caramel Coloring** – You have likely seen this ingredient often, especially if you drink soda. It is the most commonly used coloring and is found in other foods that include brown colored bread, cookies, baked good mixes, gravy, ice cream, condiments and many desserts. Caramel coloring comes from heating certain ingredients including various forms of sugar, such as fructose, sucrose or molasses as well as acids, salts and antifoaming agents. In addition, especially in the case of soda, caramel coloring includes the chemical 4-methylimidazole, which in high doses has been shown to cause cancer.

- **Castoreum** – This ingredient, which comes from the castor sacs of a beaver, is used in fruit flavored foods, especially strawberry and raspberry flavored items. On food labels, it is considered a natural ingredient, which means that those foods that claim to be "all natural" could contain parts of a beaver that you do not even want to think about!

- **Corn by-products** – Corn as a whole ingredient, such as right off of the cob, is healthy to eat. It is the additives that are derived by corn that are unhealthy. These foods are typically used as fillers in food to help them taste better or last longer, but in the end, they provide empty calories. Unfortunately it is not very easy to decipher which ingredients are by-products of corn. Some of the most common ingredients include high fructose corn syrup, xylitol, sucrose, corn oil, dextrin, dextrose, monosodium glumate, sorbitol and starch.

- **Soy By-Products** – Soy is another misleading ingredient in many products because soy is often related to healthy foods. It is the genetically processed (created in a lab) foods that are harmful. These ingredients include soybean oil, hydrolyzed soy protein, soy nuts, hydrolyzed vegetable protein and soy lecithin. In its whole form, soy can be healthy, in very small amounts. In its processed form, soy can cause hormonal issues in everyone from children to seniors and should be avoided. Unfortunately, it is found in almost every processed product as it has many benefits for stability, longevity and taste.

- **Monosodium Glumate** – This ingredient, most popularly recognized for its use in Chinese food, has a bad rap too. The studies are still out concerning its effect on one's health, but in general it is known to cause migraines, nausea, weakness and even chest pains. Typically you can recognize it by its full name or MSG, but it is sometimes hidden as hydrolyzed soy protein and autolyzed yeast.

- **Artificial Coloring** – Almost all processed foods contain some type of artificial coloring. It is obvious in some foods, including brightly colored cereals and drinks, but you might be surprised to hear about some of the other foods that contain it. Artificial coloring is used for obvious reasons, to add color to foods to make them look more appealing, but they can also be used to help a food maintain its natural color. In previous years, natural food products were used to create colors in food. Recently, however, companies have turned to colors created in a lab, which has caused concern for consumers. Many of the dyes that have been used in the past were derived from coal tar and contained highly toxic materials in them. But there are still 7 dyes that are acceptable for use in the United States. They are Blue #1, Blue #2, Green #3, Red #3, Red #40, Yellow #5 and Yellow #6. The studies are not yet conclusive on how the dyes affect humans, especially children, but there is speculation that a majority of the dyes can seriously affect the hyperness and level of attention in many children

.

- **Artificial flavors** – The word artificial pretty much says it all when it comes to food. If you are trying to clean up your diet, the word artificial should not have a place in it. Artificial flavors are chemically derived in a lab. They could be made thousands of different ways, but the common factor is that they are artificial and filled with chemicals that are harmful to your body.

These ingredients that should be avoided might have you wondering why they are allowed to be used in the food that we eat. Unfortunately, these ingredients are considered GRAS or Generally Recognized as Safe. Just because the FDA says something could potentially be safe does not mean that it is good for you and your family. It is up to you, as the decision maker in your family, to decide what is safe for your family to consume. Relying on the regulations set forth by anyone else could put the health and welfare of your family at risk.

Looking At An Example

If you are still unsure about what you should be feeding your family, let's take a look at a commonly eaten food in most households – bread. A bread that claims to be "high in fiber" might catch your eye – making you think that it is healthy. Unless that bread that is made with 100 percent whole grains, it is not high in fiber. Most breads contain the ingredient enriched wheat, unbleached wheat flour or even multigrain as one of the first ingredients. Guess what? These are not "real" wheat flours. These breads contain grains that have been stripped of their nutrients. There might be a little fiber added back with other ingredients, but it is not nearly as healthy as eating the whole grain. In addition, many breads contain several different types of sugar. Sugar is not a necessary ingredient in bread, except for the minimal amount that is necessary to activate the yeast. Corn syrup, especially high fructose corn syrup, is not necessary for bread to taste good, but it does help the shelf life, which is what makes food manufacturers use it.

We still are not done! There could also be artificial coloring, caramel coloring, corn by-products and soy by-products.

This is just one example of food that makes the claim to be healthy, but in reality is the furthest thing from healthy. As you learn how to read ingredients, you will get a thorough understanding of what you are feeding your family and how to avoid the unnecessary additives. The breads that contain added sugars, little fiber and very few vitamins are really just empty calories. They fill your stomach, but they do not provide your body with any benefits.

You Have Power

You have the power to keep the health of you and your family under control. By reading and understanding the ingredients in the food that you and your family eat, you can help everyone fight chronic diseases, control their hormones, watch their weight and even control their behavior. It sounds too good to be true, doesn't it? It is not though. The ingredient list is labeled on foods for a reason. They are there to help you know what you are eating. Just as you would follow a recipe at home, you should do the same with the food that you purchase. It is no different, except for the fact that someone else has prepared it. Do you really want to put someone else in charge of your family's health? Any food that has more than one ingredient deserves extensive scrutiny on your part. Starting at the top, take a close look at those ingredients that have the highest concentration in your food; but do not stop there. Remember that sugar can show up in many different names, meaning that each could be found in small quantities, but when you add them together – the total is huge.

The ingredients that should be avoided at all costs have been noted in this chapter, but there are thousands of ingredients that should be avoided. Remember that if you do not recognize it, do not eat it until you do your research. It is likely that you will be very surprised at the foods that you have been allowing your family to eat, but there is always room for change. Education is the first step to making positive changes in everyone's life.

Chapter 4 – What are GMOs?

Another hot topic related to clean eating that you might hear a lot about is GMOs. While you might make a conscious effort to purchase foods that say "Made without GMOs" on the front of the package, which seems to be popping up more frequently lately, you should have a thorough understanding of what they are in order to make the appropriate choices for you and your family. This is especially important in light of what we have learned thus far that what the package label says is not always what you expect it to mean.

What Are Gmos?

GMO stands for genetically modified organisms. Those words right there probably make you want to stop in your tracks. Who wants to eat foods that have been genetically modified? Unfortunately, most processed foods have a genetically modified component. These plant or animal organisms are created in a lab by using biotechnology and merging the DNA of different species. You can think of it as a crossbreeding of sorts. The most common crops to be affected by genetic modification are soy, corn and cotton. Since a majority of the processed foods that are available in the grocery store include one of these three ingredients, chances are you are consuming GMOs.

What does it mean to modify corn? In some instances, it is injected with a pesticide while in other instances it is injected with other components that make it resistant to weeds, insects and other damage. By providing this crossbreeding, farmers are able to save more money by reducing the amount of crops that they lose. But the damage does not stop there. Even if you do not consume products made with corn or corn by-products, if you eat meat, you could be consuming GMOs because the animals that your meat came from could have been fed the GMO food. The cycle is literally endless when it comes to being exposed to GMOs.

Beware Of Corn And Soy

As if it is not bad enough to think that some of the processed foods that you or your family have consumed have been modified, according to the USDA, more than 85 percent of corn is genetically modified. Going back to the last chapter where we looked at the different names of corn, you will see just how many products you have consumed that contain GMOs. Any product that contains high fructose corn syrup, xylitol, sucrose, corn oil, dextrin, dextrose, monosodium glumate, sorbitol, corn meal, corn flour and corn starch could have been modified, putting your family at risk.

The same story is true for soy products. Because cross pollination has become so popular, it is becoming increasingly difficult for farmers to find pure seeds to grow. In fact, some farmers are even looking to farm outside of the United States for this reason. In many European countries, GMO crops have been banned. With more than 90 percent of soy undergoing some type of processing, any products that contain any type of hydrogenated oils, lecithin, including soy lecithin or emulsifiers are at risk for being a GMO product.

What You Feed Your Kids

Unfortunately, the most popular products for kids, including most cereals, granola bars, cookies and crackers contain these ingredients that are at high risk for being contaminated. There is no certain way to tell if the products that your kids are eating are among the contaminated group, but is it worth the risk? In general, your best bet is to choose certified organic food. In order for a food to be considered organic by the USDA, all precautions need to have taken place to avoid the use of GMO seeds, cows can only be fed organic food and any equipment that is used can only be used on organic products to avoid cross contamination.

Where to Look

Your head is likely spinning at this point. What is left for you to eat? It seems like every food has some type of contamination in it. If you are going to continue purchasing prepackaged food, these following ingredients are the most harmful and have the highest risk at being a GMO ingredient:

- Aspartame

- Ascorbic Acid
- Citric Acid
- Any type of Flavorings
- High Fructose Corn Syrup
- MSG
- Sucrose
- Xanthan Gum
- Yeast Ingredients
- Vitamin C

Unfortunately the list does not stop there; the list continues with many more foods including Hawaiian papayas, some zucchini, vegetable oil and even some cheese. In addition to corn and soy products, you should be on the lookout for foods that contain cottonseed oil, sugar beets, alfalfa or canola. While it is virtually impossible to avoid all GMOs because there are no strict standards requiring their labeling, there are a few simple ways that you can ensure that you minimize your consumption as much as possible.

- Any sugar that is in the products that you eat should be from cane sugar, not beet sugar in order to avoid GMOs.

- If you choose organic products, make sure that they are 100 percent organic. Simply stating that a product is organic does not mean that all of the ingredients are organic; it could mean a slight fraction is organic. Instead, choose products that are certified 100 percent organic, which means that they have been approved by the USDA.

- The words "Non GMO Project Verified" will allow you to know that there are no GMOs in any given product. This labeling is becoming easier to find in your regular grocery store.

- If you are dining out, find out what type of oil that the restaurant uses to make their food. If they use corn or canola oil, they could contain GMOs.

How To Feed Your Family

Now that you know what is in the foods that you and your family have been eating, you might wonder what is left for everyone to eat. Luckily, there is plenty! It all comes back to incorporating clean eating into everyone's diet. If you have already made the pledge to ditch the processed food in your house, you have a head start on everyone else. Even if you are taking baby steps, removing one thing at a time; every step that you take is one step closer to good health for you and your family.

As you begin to remove processed products from your home, slowly introduce new products to replace the processed products. This will help to alleviate some of the angst that your family members experience as a food that they have loved and eaten for years is removed from the home.

This is not a change that is going to happen overnight, but as you slowly change the foods that you eat, everyone will start to feel healthy and enjoy what they are eating. As you learn to read more ingredients, you will come to the realization that we have all been duped by the food manufacturers. There are a large amount of chemicals and toxins in the foods that are on the market that we do not even realize. Every day new discoveries are made and another food is either modified or taken off of the shelf.

Unfortunately in the United States it is very difficult to determine which foods contain GMOs and which do not, unless they carry the "Non GMO Project Verified" label. We are one of the last countries to require food manufacturers to label products that contain GMO ingredients.

At this point it is up to the consumer to determine if a food is healthy enough for your family or not. As a nation, everyone is working together to provide more transparency for consumers to allow them to understand the products that they are eating. Until then, it is up to us to control what ingredients enter our family's bodies.

There is no cut and dry answer as of yet regarding what GMOs do to our bodies and whether or not we should avoid them. The fact that many other countries have banned them from their foods leads the way to assume that we too should do our best to avoid them. As we move through the chapters in this book and you start eliminating processed foods from your diet, it will become second nature to avoid GMOs and soon it will occur without very much effort at all. For the moment, focus on what you can change today and work your way up from there to get your family on the right track to optimal health.

Chapter 5 – Ditch the White Bread Habit

The title of this chapter just might have you groaning, especially if you have kids. How are you ever going to get them to switch from white bread to healthy bread? The color alone turns many kids off – but it is not as hard as it seems. With a little dedication, you can get kids to switch! If you are worried about how everyone will react, you certainly do not have to start with changing your bread, but you should keep it near the beginning of your plans as you begin to instill clean eating within your family.

The Misconception

One misconception that many people fall into is thinking that the bread that they are eating is healthy. Surprise! Most breads are not healthy. You are likely wondering why, just like most of us did when we realized that the bread that our families were consuming was not as healthy as we thought. You can start things off by reading the ingredients on the bread that your family normally consumes. A few of the ingredients might pop out at you now that you have learned how to read labels.

Do you see high fructose corn syrup, enriched flour, soy lecithin, corn by-products or one of the many names for sugar in the bread? Now, count how many ingredients are in that bread. Many brands have more than 35 ingredients!

If you have ever made bread from scratch, you know that you only need a handful of ingredients to make it, so why do the commercial breads have so many ingredients? The reasons vary, but they boil down to creating a longer shelf life, better (aka sweeter) taste and lower costs to make them, all of which benefit the food companies.

Another misconception that people fall for when consuming bread is the vast number of vitamins that seem to be in the bread. Even white bread can seem healthy if you are looking at vitamin content alone, but now that you understand how to read labels, you know the truth. White bread is not healthy; the vitamins and nutrients that the label claims are in the bread are added back into the bread to make them look better to consumers, but they are not nearly as healthy as the true whole grain breads.

When vitamins are added back in, they have a fraction of the health benefits of the whole grains as well as a much larger percentage of sugar and other harmful additives to help them taste good.

Choosing The Right Bread

So how do you choose the right bread? It is not as hard as you think. Follow these simple steps and you will be well on your way to purchasing only healthy, wholesome bread!

- **Don't fall for the "nine grain or multi-grain" trick.** Take a close look at the ingredients to ensure that the bread is made from 100 percent whole grain. This means that it is made from the entire kernel, not just the starchy portion, known as the endosperm. You need that bran and germ to get the nutrients from the right place. Look for ingredients such as whole wheat, whole oat or whole rye. If the word "whole" is not there, do not buy it.

- **Avoid enriched flours.** We already touched on this point, but it is worth saying again. Steer clear of any ingredients that say enriched.

- **Avoid "made with whole grains" products.** It is a trick that food manufacturers use to make you feel good about the bread that you are purchasing. You walk away thinking that you are eating bread made with whole grains and that you are doing your body good. While this might be true, what they are neglecting to say is that it is also made with partial grains and enriched ingredients.

- **Look for special ingredients**. When you eat whole grain bread you are not stuck with a life of boring, whole grain bread. Whole grain can actually taste delicious, especially when your favorite seeds or nuts are added in for texture and flavor. Just make sure those ingredients are wholesome.

Getting Kids To Switch

Now comes the hard part. You know what bread that your family should be eating; now how do you get them to eat it? If you have been feeding everyone white bread for years, it might be intimidating to suggest that they try something different. It is not impossible though! Here are a few simple tricks that can work on kids and those grown-up kids too:

- **Take things slow** – We have always said since the beginning of this book that you need to make slow changes. This is very true when switching to whole grain bread. If your kids are resistant, start by making half of the sandwich whole grain and the other half their old standby white bread. This allows kids to have the comfort of having their "old" bread with their sandwich, while giving them the benefit of trying whole grain bread.

- **Get creative** – Kids love when their food takes on different shapes or patterns. Let loose and have fun with their sandwiches. You can use cookie cutters to make fun shapes or make faces on the top of the bread with cherry tomatoes, olives, cucumbers and any other foods that your kids like and will not turn their nose up at.

- **Make your own** – Bread making is not as intimidating as it sounds. Once you make your first loaf, chances are you will be hooked. Before you do though, let the kids get in the kitchen with you. Let them see the difference between white flour and whole grain flour. Let them get their hands dirty and knead the dough. When they are a part of the action, they are more likely to want to eat it.

- **Educate your kids** – Let your kids know why you are making the switch and why you think that they should too. When kids have an understanding of what they are eating, they might surprise you and willingly switch to whole grain bread.

- Make it fun – Let your kids help you grocery shop and put them on the hunt for whole grain bread. Teach them the difference between whole grain and enriched grains and see which breads they come up with that they think are healthy. Make it like a scavenger hunt in the store and your kids are more likely to be excited about it.

Moving Beyond Bread

Unfortunately, white bread is not the only unhealthy grain you might be consuming. Do you consume white pasta and white rice? If you do, then you have more work to do. Luckily, changing over foods such as pasta and rice is not as difficult as switching bread. You can get creative with your pastas and rice to disguise the change and encourage everyone to eat healthy. If you want to start simple, swap white rice for brown rice and whole grain pasta for white pasta. The taste is pretty similar and can even be masked with the addition of veggies or a homemade sauce. As everyone's taste buds begin to expand, you can get a little more adventurous with the whole grains, adding unique items such as barley, millet and quinoa to your meals.

If you make a lot of baked goods, slowly begin to adapt them by swapping out half of the white flour for whole wheat flour. As you begin to get used to the taste, you can experiment a little more. It is important to know that whole grain flours are denser than white flour, so it might be necessary to adjust the recipes a little bit. One of the best ways to adjust them is to bake the items in smaller portions, such as making muffins instead of bread or mini sized muffins instead of traditional size.

This will cut down on the baking time and ensure that the items bake all the way through. Eventually you will want to swap out your recipes for whole grain versions. Chances are that most of the baked goods that you make have a healthy alternative that will satisfy cravings yet be a little healthier.

Cooking With Grains

If you want to begin adding grains to your dinner table, there are so many to choose from. In general, it is very easy to cook grains; even those that you have never heard of can be cooked fairly easy. The biggest concern is the amount of time that they take. In general, to cook any grain, you put it in the pan and cover it with enough water to touch the top of the grain. You then bring the water to a boil, lower it to simmer and let the grains cook until the water is absorbed. If you feel as if your grains are not tender enough when the water has absorbed, simply add more water and let them cook longer.

If you do not have time to let the grains get as tender as you like, there are a few shortcuts to take:

- **Cook your grains in large batches at the beginning of the week** – If you meal plan, this can be a great time saver. Cooking your grains on Sunday or Monday allows you to enjoy them all week long. You can use them as dinner side dishes, main dishes or even as additions to your lunch. Quinoa, bulgur and brown rice all make wonderful bases for salads.

- **Presoak your grains** – If you do not want to make big batches, another shortcut is to soak your grains ahead of time. Usually letting any grain soak in the same amount of water that you would cook them in for a few hours drastically cuts down the cooking time. When you are ready to cook the grains, simply add more water to the pan and get them cooking.

The best way to get kids excited about eating whole grain breads, pastas and rice is to get them involved in the kitchen with you. Let kids help you find recipes and create them. They will be proud to show off their hard work and much more likely to give the new items a try. Remember to take things slow and do not push the new healthier grains on anyone; as we all know, food that is pushed onto kids will be more likely to be resisted. Make it as fun as possible, creating funny shapes and patterns whenever you can to help kids want to eat healthy and think that it is fun!

Chapter 6 – Ditch the Fast Food

When you have a busy family, it usually means that there is no time for eating. We have all been there. Everyone comes to sit at the table and different times. Some family members do not even make it to the table, they end up eating on the go, whether in the car or at their practice or wherever their activities take them. Sometimes, probably more often than you would like to admit, your lunches and/or dinners are handed to you from a fast food window. This is the habit that we need to put an end to, no matter how difficult it may seem. The first few weeks of "just saying no to fast food," will be a major change, but in a matter of a few days to a few weeks, it will become much easier. The key is in proper planning, which we will discuss.

Time is Valuable

Many people fall into the fast food trap because they think that they do not have time to cook. What they seem to forget is that going to the fast food restaurant, waiting in line, ordering, paying, waiting for your food and taking it home takes up TIME too! When you think of it that way, you might just have more time to cook than you originally thought. Not every meal has to be a "gourmet" meal served with linen napkins and several courses. Instead, with the help of your family, you can come up with a list of "fast meals" meaning those meals that take 20 minutes or less to put together but are much healthier than the "mystery nuggets" coming from the drive thru.

Unfair Marketing

Unfortunately, you have the unfair marketing practices that food companies use to lure kids into wanting their food. It is not just on television that these ads are being seen either. Kids are exposed to ads online, in video games, at the movie theater and in many other merchandising methods. Just look at the large number of very young children that can recognize the logo of fast food restaurants well before they are able to read. The marketing is out there and it definitely makes it difficult for parents to keep their kids on track with healthy eating.

Educate your Kids

Chances are your kids, just like most kids, are not going to take the news that they cannot have their favorite chicken nuggets or French fries anymore very easily. This is yet another habit that you will have to slowly stop. The best way to start it off is by educating your kids about fast food. No matter how young or old they are, they can learn an age appropriate lesson about the food that is served at these restaurants and how it does not do them any good. You do not have to become a preacher and constantly harp on your kids about the nutrition in food, but you can use it as a lesson every so often to help them understand how fast food contains very few nutrients that are good for their bodies.

You could also show them how you can make healthier alternatives at home. Chicken nuggets that are sold in most drive-thru windows are not whole pieces of chicken, but rather are the scraps of skin, carcass and other parts that you would rather not think about. At home, you can make a much healthier and better tasting version that your kids will love! The same is true for burgers, French fries and many other fast food favorites.

You Are The Role Model

If there is one thing that we know about kids, it is that they follow whatever we do. If you make it a habit to swing through the drive thru on a busy day, then the kids are going to start expecting that for them as well. If instead, you head home and make one of your "quick" meals and enjoy a healthy meal of low fat protein, fruits and vegetables, your kids will come to see that as the normal, healthy habit that they should have as well.

Remember that this change is not going to happen overnight and your kids are not going to jump up and down with excitement when they learn that fast food is not going to be your go-to meal on busy nights, but it will become easier with time. On nights that you have more time, make the fast food meals at home that your kids love. Instead of serving a burger with fattening oil soaked French fries, serve it with a healthy salad or beautiful fruit salad. If your kids really miss the French fries, you can bake your own without the oil and skip the frying.

Keep Kids Full

Another key factor in helping kids and adults, for that matter, ditch the fast food habit is to keep everyone full.

That does not mean to gorge on any food that you want. It means eating the right foods at the right times and always having snacks on hand. Think back to the last five times that you went to the local fast food restaurant and the reasons that you went.

Did one or more of your reasons include the fact that the kids were starving and whining in the backseat because they had gone from one activity to another or one errand to the next without anything to eat? When blood sugar levels get low enough, everyone can get whiny and desperate for whatever food is available.

Rather than letting that happen, always be prepared. Portion out healthy snacks that are portable, such as grapes, carrots, celery, popcorn, rice cakes or nuts. Keep travel size bags in your car or purse and be ready to dole them out when the kids are getting hungry. Now instead of dragging around crabby, hungry kids that whine for every fast food drive thru that they see, you will have satisfied, happy kids that are less likely to beg for fast food.

Make Kid Friendly Food

Those days that your kids really want chicken nuggets, French fries or other fast food type food, you can help by being ready with kid friendly clean eating recipes. No, they will not likely look the same as the fast food version and honestly, who wants it to look like that anyways? What matters is how they taste and as far as everyone is concerned, the clean eating version is so much better. Unfortunately today, most kids are so used to the fast food versions that it is what they think is actually good. Once they are given the taste of "real" food that truly tastes good, the fast food suddenly will not taste so good anymore.

What can you make at home that will rival the best fast food out there? Here are just a few of the options:

- Tacos
- Burgers
- Chicken nuggets or chicken fingers
- French fries
- Salads
- Wraps

You might still be in denial, so let's take a look at what clean eating chicken nuggets for kids would look like. You might not believe it, but chicken nuggets really only need three ingredients: chicken breasts, whole wheat bread crumbs and egg whites. The egg whites are what bind the bread crumbs to the chicken pieces. That's it!

The best part about this recipe is that you can make your own breadcrumbs and customize them to your own preferences. Breadcrumbs can be made in large batches, which mean that you can make them whenever you have time and store them in an airtight container in the refrigerator for a week or in the freezer for up to 6 months!

If your kids like a little kick in their chicken nuggets, use chili powder or cumin to spice things up. If they prefer Italian style breadcrumbs, you can use garlic powder, oregano and basil for your base. To make the chicken nuggets, simply follow this recipe:

Clean Eating Fast Food Chicken Nuggets

- Chicken breasts (1/2 of a breast per person)
- Bread crumbs
- 1 egg white per chicken breast made

Whisk the eggs until they are light and fluffy. Cut the chicken breasts into bite size pieces. Roll the chicken pieces around in the egg white and then coat them with the breadcrumbs. Bake them on a flat cookie sheet prepared with olive oil at 350 degrees for 15 minutes or until cooked through.

French Fries at Home

Yes, you can still feed your kids French fries! The difference is you will make them at home without the fattening and toxin filled oils. There are several ways that you can serve French fries; you can make them with Yukon or red potatoes, making them look like the fries that kids are used to or you can substitute sweet potatoes or even green beans to give the French fry crunch but with many more nutrients. If your kids are still at the stage of turning their nose up at anything with color, go ahead and start with this basic recipe.

- Clean Eating Baked French Fries
- 2 Yukon or red potatoes scrubbed clean

- 2 teaspoons olive oil
- Salt and pepper to taste

After scrubbing your potatoes, peel them and slice them as thin as possible. If your kids love thin, crispy fries, this step is very important. After slicing them, place the potato strips in a bowl and cover with 2 teaspoons of olive oil. Stir the potatoes around until the potatoes are evenly covered and then sprinkle with salt and pepper to taste.

Place the potatoes in a thin layer on a parchment paper lined cookie sheet. Bake at 400 degrees on the bottom rack.

- A few important notes about baking fries. Make sure that the potatoes are not crowded on the cookie sheet; the more crowded they are, the more moisture that gets created, resulting in soggy fries. Keep the baking sheet as close to the bottom as possible to prevent the outside from cooking too fast and the inside remaining soggy.

- You can alter the seasonings to your family's taste preferences. Get creative with spicy spices or garlic powder and parmesan cheese.

Once you are well on your way in your endeavor to eat clean, do not be afraid to substitute sweet potatoes for the Yukon or red potatoes. You can use the same method and same spices, but get a lot more nutrients and even taste out of them. You could also try one of the below delicious recipes:

Green Bean "Fries"

- 1 pound fresh green beans, ends snipped
- 2 teaspoons olive oil (or coconut oil)
- 1/8 cup parmesan cheese
- 1 tsp garlic powder
- Sea salt to taste

Combine all ingredients in a bowl until thoroughly coated. Place in a single layer on a parchment paper lined cookie sheet and bake at 375 degrees for 15-20 minutes or until crisp.

After you get your kids or other family members used to enjoying their "fries" in the shape that they are used to, try to experiment. Believe it or not many roasted vegetables that get the same crispiness as fries do are just as satisfying and a whole lot more nutritious.

Experiment with vegetables including broccoli, asparagus and cauliflower. Each of these vegetables can be brushed with a little bit of olive or coconut oil and then seasoned with the seasonings that your family prefers. When you place the vegetables on the baking sheet, make sure to place them far apart to ensure that they have enough room to cook. Bake them until they have the desired level of crispiness of your family and enjoy!

Clean Eating Burgers

Burgers are one of the easiest fast food type foods to make at home and they are completely customizable. If your family is still trying to get used to clean eating, you can still use ground meat for your burgers; just make sure to use the leanest meat available and purchase organic or grass-fed if you can. As you make more changes, you might find that you turn to lean ground turkey or even make your own veggie patties.

The best way to ensure that your meat is clean is to avoid purchasing prepackaged meat – instead purchase from your local butcher. If you are comfortable with it, you can even ask your butcher to grind your meat for you straight from the whole meat. This way you know for sure that there are no additives or preservatives in your meat.

Once you have a clean eating meat as your base, you can make your burgers using your favorite recipe. Burgers are very forgiving and allow you to customize them however you want.

A Burger with Variety

One of the largest differences in clean eating burgers is not only the type of meat that you use, but also the binder that you use to keep the meat together.

Traditionally, burgers use breadcrumbs. You could substitute whole wheat breadcrumbs in place of white breadcrumbs or if you are feeling adventurous, you could try omitting the breadcrumbs altogether. Sometimes all that you need is an egg white or two to bind things together.

With your base of lean, organic meat, whole wheat breadcrumbs and an egg white, you can then customize your burger with spices including:

- Onion powder
- Garlic powder
- Italian seasonings
- Fresh vegetables including onions, tomatoes or garlic

The options are endless when it comes to using spices. If your family likes burgers with a kick, try adding cumin, chili powder or paprika. If they prefer things plain, just a little sea salt and pepper might do the trick.

How you top your burgers will matter too! If your kids must have a bun, forgo the $1 buns at the grocery store that are filled with high fructose corn syrup, enriched flour and plenty of other harmful ingredients. Instead, purchase whole grain buns, do without the bun or get creative and use portabella mushrooms, large lettuce leaves or thinly sliced zucchini as a bun. Your kids might think it is fun to experiment with different ways to eat their burger.

As you navigate your family's way through the clean eating diet, it will start to become second nature. Soon enough, you will be able to pass by previously favorite fast food restaurants and not have to stop. Instead you will be able to go home to a home cooked, delicious and nutritious meal that everyone can feel good about.

Chapter 7 – Learn to Try New Foods

The hardest part of instilling a clean eating diet within your family is getting everyone to try new foods. If you have kids that instantly wrinkle up their nose when something new shows up on their plate, you are not alone. Living a life on processed foods has continually trained everyone's taste buds to look for exceptionally sweet, processed tastes, making the natural, clean foods seem boring.

As you will soon learn, it is the processed foods that should be considered boring because they are stripped of all of their nutrients. The ingredients that you taste are mostly chemicals and additives, not the true taste of delicious clean eating food. Before you give up on this step of trying to introduce new foods into your family's diet, try one of the following ways to get your kids and the grownups in your house to become adventurous with the foods that they taste.

The One Bite Rule

Were you brought up in the "clean plate club"? Most of us were brought up under the notion that we had to completely clean our plates for various reasons that our parents came up with every day. Today, that is not suggested. In fact, it is suggested that we do not force or encourage our kids to eat all of the food on their plate.

Instead, we should encourage a healthy consumption of food and allow children to determine when they are full on their own. This leads us to the "One Bite rule." Under this rule, you simply encourage everyone at the table to take at least one bite of every food that is on their plate. This gives everyone a fair chance at trying a new food without forcing them to eat a large amount of something that they truly do not like.

A way to simplify the "One Bite rule" is to encourage everyone to say something about the new food after trying it. You can use this as a method to promote positive talk about new food items, rather than only negative comments that allow kids to avoid having to eat more of a food that they do not like. Let kids explore the smell, texture, look and taste of the food. Encourage your kids to discover things that they like and do not like about a food. This will give you options in the future if you decide to make the food a different way. If you do decide to use the "One Bite rule" try to remain flexible with your rule and never offer a reward for trying the new food. As kids grow up, they can begin to resent those foods that they were "rewarded" to eat. Instead, make it a family effort to try new foods together and use it as a discussion point at the dinner table. It can make dinner more fun and make trying new foods an adventure.

Get Kids in the Kitchen

We have touched on this topic a little bit before, but it is worth repeating. Get your kids in the kitchen and let them help you prepare the meals. You might wonder why this is so important. Isn't it easier to prepare meals without your kids under tow? Believe it or not, a study performed by Columbia University has shown that kids that help prepare meals are more likely to eat the foods that they prepared. This of course, is not a guarantee that kids are going to like every new food that crosses their plate, but it is a higher guarantee that they will at the very least, try the new food.

When you encourage your kids to come into the kitchen and help, make sure that you provide tasks that they can easily accomplish. You can encourage kids of all ages to help you, as long as you tailor their tasks to their abilities. Of course, you only want to do this when you are not in a crunch for time. Save the kitchen duties for weekends or days during the week that you do not have a lot of running around to do. This allows everyone to be more relaxed and have the opportunity for fun in the kitchen. If you are stressed, it will make the kids stressed and the opportunity to learn about new foods will be lost. Letting kids help in the kitchen should be a fun way to incorporate them into learning to eat healthier.

Many Preparations

Most foods have many different ways that they can be prepared. If your family turns their nose up at a new food the first time that you prepare it, try a different recipe. There are likely many different ways to make a variety of new foods, whether they are common foods, such as broccoli or a lesser known food, such as barley. The internet is a very valuable resource when it comes to preparing new foods; you can likely find hundreds of recipes for one ingredient if you search hard enough. This really comes in handy when a new food that you have introduced does not go as well as planned. You have many other opportunities to see if there is another preparation that everyone enjoys a little more.

Let's use broccoli as a simple example. Yes, most kids turn their nose up at broccoli, but they might be willing to try it if you serve it in a variety of different ways including:

- Raw with a homemade hummus or clean eating, homemade ranch dip (most kids like anything with dip)
- Steamed with a little parmesan cheese on top
- Grilled
- Sautéed in a little olive oil with a few garlic cloves
- Mixed into a green salad
- Roasted in the oven with a drizzle of olive oil and parmesan cheese

As another example, let's look at edamme:

- Shelled edamme drizzled with olive oil and sprinkled with parmesan cheese, baked at 400 degrees until crispy
- Added to a salad
- Steamed and tossed with a little olive oil and lemon juice

- Mix edamme with a whole grain, such as quinoa, and corn and drizzle with olive oil, lemon juice, lime juice and your favorite seasoning

There are no steadfast rules when it comes to preparing healthy food with the exception that you use natural, clean eating ingredients. Feel free to experiment on your own, creating your own recipes or letting the kids come up with their favorite way to prepare nutritious food to incorporate as many healthy foods into your family's life as possible.

You are the Role Model

If you expect your kids to try new foods, they will expect you to try them too. Let your kids see you eating the new food and they will likely follow suit. As you eat it, talk about it to the kids. Tell them what you like about the texture, smell, appearance and taste. Tell each of your children what you think they might like about the food and then encourage them to try it. When you make the new food more of a game rather than a chore or requirement, everyone is likely to at least give it a try. Just remember that they are watching your every move, so if you try a food that you really do not like, try to control your reaction so that the kids do not follow suit without trying the new food.

Try Not To Hide Food

Some people might try to disguise new foods by hiding them in other recipes, such as meatballs or muffins. If you want your kids to get a full appreciation of a new food, it is best not to hide it. You want your kids to see what they are eating and to know all of its benefits. As a part of a clean eating diet, your recipes will not have a large number of ingredients, which makes it more difficult to hide ingredients as it is. Instead of hiding the foods, let your kids explore them in many different ways. This allows them to get a full appreciation of the foods that they eat and to learn what keeps them healthy.

Get Creative

Let's face it, healthy food does not always look enticing to kids as is, but you can make it look enticing! Kids have a knack for getting excited about foods that are in different shapes and patterns that make food more fun.

There are no rules regarding how to make the food look fun for your kids. A few of the ways that you can use include:

- Use cookie cutters to make fun shapes
- Create faces using different types of fruits and vegetables (use some fruits/vegetables that your kids are used to and introduce a new one or two this way)
- Make flower shapes with different fruits and vegetables
- Shave the foods with a cheese grater to make them look like ribbons
- Make a rainbow of colors with many different types of food
- Make kabobs out of fruits and vegetables because everything tastes better on a stick

The key is to stay positive and offer different types of food often, not giving up after just one try. You can do your best to only offer new foods when your kids are most likely to receive them well, but you might not always hit the nail on the head. This is why it is important to keep trying. As long as you stay positive, remain a good role model for your child and continue to get creative, you will get your kids to enjoy new foods that are good for them eventually, it just might take some time.

Chapter 8 – Learn How To Snack Healthy

Snacking can be one of the hardest transitions to make when you adopt a clean eating diet in your family. Because everyone is so busy, it is easy to turn to quick, aka processed snacks, in a box, bag or some type of package. We want instant gratification and the only way that we know how to get it is with processed foods. The good news is that we can turn those habits around and it will not be as grueling as you might think. Yes, it will require a little more preparation, but before long, you will be used to it and it will no longer seem like a chore.

Snacking is Good for You

The first thing that you should understand is that snacking is good for you and your kids. It keeps blood sugar levels stable and keeps metabolism going. That being said, what you snack on greatly matters. Obviously a snack of potato chips or a candy bar is not going to do your body any good, but a snack of raw fruit, vegetables or a handful of nuts will give your body what it needs to stay fueled. The key is to focus on clean eating snacks and eating in moderation. This does not mean that your snacking is banned to apple slices and celery. There are plenty of ways to make snacking exciting without colorful packages, even for kids.

Where to Focus

Now that you have stepped away from prepackaged food, how do you grab fast snacks? You will want to put your focus on whole fruits and vegetables, whole grains and nuts. While fruits and vegetables will need to be purchased on a weekly basis in order to guarantee freshness, nuts, seeds and whole grains can be purchased in bulk and prepared ahead of time. Start by making a list of the fruits, vegetables, whole grains and nuts that your family enjoys. The next time that you grocery shop, purchase these items in bulk. Once you have a foundation to work with, you can build up from there, especially as your family's repertoire of food choices increases.

Preparation is Key

Perhaps one of the hardest parts of snacking on a clean eating diet is finding the time to get snacks prepared. The best way to do this is to set aside one day to prepare for the week. In the beginning it will take a little more time to get used to, but once you have done it for a few weeks it will become habit and get done much quicker. Pick a day that you have a little extra time and slice fruits and vegetables, placing them in individual portions that can easily be grabbed as you run out the door.

You can also create your own "packages" of nuts, seeds, air popped popcorn, unsalted whole grain rice cakes and whole grain crackers with no added ingredients. If your family loves peanut butter or other natural nut butters, make individual portions of these "dips" and put them alongside your apple, banana and celery slices for an extra kick of protein and a good filler.

These are just a sample of the "quick" snacks that you can put together. When you have a little more time on your hands, you can create the following snacks. Each of them will keep in the refrigerator for a week or so, which allows you to make them once and have snacks ready during the busiest part of your week.

Remember the Crispy Edamme from the previous chapter? Those make great on-the-go snacks. Make a big batch and package them individually for a fun treat throughout the week. Pop a large batch of popcorn and portion it out for grabbing throughout the week. To make your popcorn even healthier, skip the stove top and pop it in the microwave in a brown paper bag!

Now you have the convenience of microwave popcorn without all of the unnecessary ingredients that are harmful to your body. You can season your popcorn however everyone likes it, but the best news is that you do not need to use oil or salt.

Try seasonings such:

- Parmesan cheese
- A couple of sprays of olive oil and parmesan cheese
- A couple of sprays of olive oil and Italian seasoning
- Chili powder
- A couple of sprays of olive oil and tabasco sauce
- A tablespoon of melted (real) butter with cinnamon and a tiny bit of real sugar

Hummus

Homemade hummus is another great dip to keep handy. It goes well with almost any vegetable and can make snacking just a little more fun, plus you get the added benefit of more nutrients because hummus is made with delicious, yet healthy chick peas. You can start with a basic hummus recipe and then begin adding spices as you see fit down the road.

Basic Hummus Recipe

- 1 can chickpeas
- 1/8 cup olive oil
- 2 teaspoons fresh lemon juice
- ½ teaspoon cumin or paprika (depending on your family's preference)

Place all ingredients in a food processor or blender and blend until smooth.

If your family is a bit more adventurous, you can add many different types of ingredients to the basic hummus recipe such as fresh jalapenos, cilantro, lime juice, mint, basil, dill and even black beans or artichokes for a little more texture. There are no steadfast rules for hummus. Once you have mastered the basic recipe, feel free to experiment with different tastes to see what your family likes. Hummus is a wonderful addition to raw vegetables or even whole grain pitas.

The Versatility of Peanut Butter

Peanut butter is one of those things that goes good on almost anything! That is why it is important to have a large stash of it around the house all of the time; it can literally take any snack from boring to exciting in seconds. If your family adores peanut butter and does not have any allergies – have fun with these recipes! It is recommended that you use natural peanut butter as many brands of "regular" peanut butter contain trans-fat and other additives that just are not necessary in peanut butter. If you do have peanut allergies or an aversion to peanut butter, any type of natural nut butter that is tolerated will also work.

Peanut Butter Yogurt Dip

- ¾ cup natural Greek Yogurt (plain)
- ½ cup natural peanut butter (or any other nut butter)
- 1 tsp honey (use raw honey whenever possible; honey is also optional)
- Cinnamon to taste
- ½ teaspoon vanilla

Mix all ingredients with a hand mixer until perfectly smooth. Refrigerate for 2 hours before eating. This dip goes perfect with any type of fruit including a variety of apples and sliced bananas.

If you are in a time crunch and do not have any of this dip on hand, you can use straight, natural peanut butter on foods including:

- Apples
- Celery
- Bananas
- Whole grain crackers
- Whole grain bread (toasted)

For your family members that need a little more crunch, natural granola can add a wonderful taste. Spread granola over your apple and peanut butter or banana and peanut butter for a delicious, nutritious and filling snack!

Homemade Granola

If you have not tried making your own granola yet, it is worth a try. It is not as overwhelming as it seems and can really add to the excitement of your family's snacks. The largest benefit of making your own granola is that you get to control the ingredients that go into it, including the amount of sugar as well as the additions, in order to tailor them to what your family likes. Granola can keep for quite a while in an airtight container, which makes it easy to make large batches at a time, allowing your family to enjoy this healthy snack without a lot of blood, sweat and tears from you.

Homemade Granola Options

The basis of homemade granola is "real" oats. This does not mean the quick cook or instant oats you find in the breakfast aisle at the grocery store. You want the whole oat, which means that you are giving your family the entire grain and lots of nutrition! You can still find whole oats in the same aisle as the quick cook oats or to save money, you can buy them in bulk at many stores. In addition to oats, the rest is up to you and what your family likes. You will need a "wet" ingredient which could be any of the following:

- Coconut oil
- Macadamia nut oil
- Natural peanut butter
- Unsweetened applesauce
- Pure pumpkin puree

You only need as much of the "wet" ingredient as is necessary to moisten the oats and make all of your ingredients stick together or become moistened.

You can add any of the following ingredients, again, according to your family's preferences:

- Raw nuts (any variety)
- Dried fruit (make sure it is unsweetened and use sparingly)
- Unsweetened coconut
- Any type of seeds
- Cinnamon
- Pumpkin spice
- Vanilla extract
- Almond extract
- Raw honey (if you need to add a little sweetness)

All that you need to do is mix your oats, wet ingredients and mix-ins together until completely coated. Spread the mixture onto a baking sheet and bake at 350 degrees for 30-45 minutes, turning the granola over every ten minutes to prevent burning.

Homemade Trail Mix

Another popular snack that gets a bad rap is trail mix and for good reason. Prepackaged trail mix contains a large amount of trans fat, sugar and unnecessary additives. This does not mean that your family is banned from this beloved snack now that you have started a clean eating lifestyle. Instead, in your preparations, you can make a large batch of healthy trail mix that will last your family a few weeks and will keep everyone happy and healthy! Trail mix is one of the more popular snacks to prepare and keep around because it is very portable and delicious. The key to making a good trail mix is getting creative. Think about the things that your family likes – do they love coconut? Then make a trail mix with a Hawaiian flair. If they love nuts, seeds or raisins, make sure to include those. Just be mindful of the sugar content in any ingredients that you add in, always opting for the unsweetened or no-sugar-added version.

Almost anything goes when you make your own trail mix, but here are a few ideas to use in your next batch:

- Unsweetened coconut
- Any type of raw nuts
- No sugar added raisins or other dried fruit
- Seeds (especially pumpkin or sunflower)
- Toasted whole oats
- No sugar added Goji berries
- Hemp seeds
- Dark chocolate chips (use sparingly and purchase raw chocolate nibs if possible)
- Any type of spices including spicy, sweet or a combination of both

Homemade Ranch Dip

Just like peanut butter, ranch dip seems to make everything taste better, especially for kids. As you guessed, the store bought version contains unnecessary sugar and additives. It is fairly easy to whip up your own batch. The ingredients are much simpler than you would probably guess and you might even have them lying around your house!

One of the fastest ways to get your ranch dressing fix is to make your own ranch dressing spices, you know the type that you can purchase in the packet yet has chemicals that you do not even want to think about in them. This way you have the spices ready and all that you have to do is add your Greek yogurt and refrigerate for a few hours and you have your own, homemade clean eating Ranch dressing!

Ranch Dressing Mix

- 1 ½ teaspoon Dill spice
- 1 teaspoon Garlic powder
- 1 teaspoon Parmesan cheese
- ½ teaspoon Onion powder
- 1 ½ teaspoon Dried parsley
- Salt and pepper to taste

To make this into a dressing, simple combine 1 tablespoon of your dressing mix with 1/3 cup of Greek yogurt and 1/3 cup of low-fat milk or buttermilk. Add the milk in slowly, judging its consistency before using the entire amount.

** If you are making the Ranch dressing to eat fresh, you can replace the garlic powder with fresh, minced garlic. ***Each of these spices can be altered to account for your family's preferences.

Delicious Frozen Fruit

For some reason everything tastes better cold for kids, even fruit! Experiment with various types of fruit and ways to freeze them. For example, grapes taste just like a delicious popsicle when frozen. Simply wash your grapes, dry them thoroughly and place them on a cookie sheet in the freezer. Once frozen, they can be placed in a container together and enjoyed!

Berries also taste delicious frozen, but to add an even more nutritious punch to them, add Greek yogurt!

- Greek Yogurt Frozen Berries
- 1 package fresh, organic raspberries or blueberries
- 1 individual container of plain Greek yogurt
- Raw honey to taste if needed

After washing and thoroughly drying your berries, dip them in the Greek Yogurt (using a toothpick is the easiest). Place them in an even layer on a parchment paper lined cookie sheet and freeze them for at least one hour. Once they are frozen, you can individually package them for snacks-on-the-go.

Miscellaneous Snacks to Have on Hand

In addition to those snacks that you prepare, you can have a variety of other snacks to have on hand all of the time including:

- Greek yogurt (throw in some healthy berries or your homemade granola)
- Any type of fruit sliced up
- Shelled edamme (eaten plain)
- Cucumbers, carrots, celery sliced up
- Raw broccoli or cauliflower (kids love ranch dip with this)
- Brown rice Rice Cakes
- Whole grain crackers
- Whole grain bread
- Whole wheat tortillas (spread with hummus and veggies)
- Unsweetened apple sauce (top with cinnamon)
- Berries

As you can see, snacking is not as hard as it seems even when clean eating. With a little preparation and the right foods bought from the grocery store, you and your family can snack healthy without consuming processed, chemically filled foods!

Chapter 9 - Recipes for Delicious Breakfasts, Lunches and Dinners on a Clean Eating Diet

Now that you have a few ways to get your family onto a clean eating diet, no matter how busy you might be, it is time to put a few more recipes to the test. Remember that even if your family turns their nose up at one preparation of clean eating food, do not give up. Try different preparations, as many as 5-10 times to see if there is another way that your family will enjoy the food. The most important factor is to have fun! Cooking and eating as a family should be fun and lighthearted, not stressful.

Breakfast

Breakfast is one of those meals that everyone tends to rush through. In fact, many people even skip it, which is the worst thing that you can do for your body, whether you are a child or adult. With a little preparation, it can be easy to serve clean eating breakfast options that do not make your morning even more stressful than it might already be on most days. As you move your family through the clean eating diet, you will want to start eliminating boxed cereal as your "go-to" food. You will also want to eliminate those convenient store bought muffins, biscuits and sandwiches that pop into the microwave and are ready to go in less than one minute. The good news is that you can prepare all of these items on your own, ahead of time and make it easy to eat clean on the go!

Breakfast Recipes

Smoothies are a fantastic way to start everyone's day off right. The best thing about smoothies is that you can customize them to fit everyone's tastes and/or needs. This basic smoothie recipe will get you started and then you can customize however you see fit:

Basic Smoothie Starter:

- 1 cup plain Greek yogurt (no added sugar)
- ½ cup strawberries hulled and sliced
- ½ banana sliced
- Small amount of raw honey if needed for sweetness

Beyond the basics of strawberries and banana, you can add any type of fruit or even veggies that you want! A few great ideas include:

- Peanut butter
- Mangoes
- Pears
- Pineapple
- Blueberries
- Raspberries
- Spinach
- Chard
- Kale
- Carrots
- Flax seeds
- Ground whole oats
- Cinnamon
- Wheat germ

Use any of these ingredients in any combination and have fun experimenting with different, delicious tastes!

Yogurt Parfaits

If you need a way to make yogurt more exciting, make a parfait out of them. Kids will look at them like they are dessert and just might complain a little less when you serve them in the morning.

- Plain Greek yogurt
- Strawberries/Blueberries/Raspberries
- Whole, raw nuts, such as walnuts or almonds
- Homemade granola

Layer the ingredients any way that you would like or let the kids make their own creations.

Pancakes With No Flour

Pancakes are a staple in many homes, especially those with kids. Eating clean does not mean that you have to give up this delicious morning breakfast, but you might want to try a new recipe or two to make them a little cleaner. Did you know it was possible to make pancakes without flour? In this recipe, bananas make up the bulk of the pancake and they taste wonderful!

Delicious Banana Pancakes

- 2 overripe bananas mashed
- 3 eggs
- 1 egg white
- ½ cup oats
- ½ teaspoon baking powder
- 1 teaspoon cinnamon
- ½ teaspoon vanilla

Place all of the ingredients in a blender and blend until completely smooth. If the batter seems too runny, gradually add a little more oats until you reach the desired consistency. Then cook the batter as you normally would cook your pancakes and serve! If you want to add a little sweetness, you can top with blueberries or strawberries and omit the need for syrup.

Baked Oatmeal

Sometimes getting kids to eat a bowl of delicious oatmeal is not an easy task. Other days, there is just no time to sit and eat it. This does not mean that you have to forget about the valuable nutrition that oatmeal provides. Instead, make oatmeal cupcakes that can be eaten on the go. Besides, what kid will argue with a "cupcake" for breakfast?

Oatmeal Cupcakes

- 1 egg
- 1 ½ teaspoons vanilla extract
- 1 cup applesauce, unsweetened
- ½ cup banana, mashed
- 1/4 cup raw honey
- 2 3/4 cups whole oats
- 2 ½ teaspoons ground cinnamon (more or less to taste)
- 1 1/2 teaspoon baking powder
- pinch of salt
- 1 1/4 cups organic milk

Mix the first 5 ingredients well. Add the oats, cinnamon, baking powder and salt, stirring until completely combined. Add the milk last. Line a muffin pan with cupcake liners and pour the batter until each liner is 2/3rds full. Once full, you can customize each "cupcake" with a variety of toppings including:

- Raw nuts
- Blueberries
- Raspberries
- Raisins
- Flax seeds

Bake at 350 for 25 minutes or until cooked through. Once cooled, you can freeze them individually for quick morning breakfasts that pop right into the microwave for less than one minute!

Quick Breakfasts

Of course not everyone has the time every morning to prepare a full breakfast or you tire of the on the go stuff. In these cases, take out your healthiest whole grain bread and make the following fun breakfasts:

Avocado Toast – It might sound odd, but freshly made guacamole spread on healthy, whole grain toast is not only delicious, but incredibly healthy.

Guacamole is not as time consuming to make as it might sound and it can be prepared at the beginning of the week. It will last for a few days as long as it is stored with plastic wrap directly on top of the guacamole, preventing any air from getting to it to cause it to turn brown.

- Guacamole Recipe
- 2 ripe avocados (insides scooped out)
- ½ of a lemon (squeezed for the juice)
- 2 teaspoons garlic powder
- 1 ½ teaspoons onion powder
- Pinch of salt

Mash all ingredients together and store in the refrigerator for use throughout the week.

Peanut Butter Toast – Spread all natural peanut butter or any other natural nut butter on toast for a wholesome breakfast.

Peanut Butter Toast with Fruit – If you want a little extra kick, top your peanut butter toast with sliced bananas and a little flax seed

Lunch

Lunch might make you a little nervous when you start eating clean, but rest assured there are plenty of ways to serve delicious lunch that will make everyone forget about drive-thrus and packaged lunch meat. The bulk of the work to make clean eating lunches can be done in the beginning of the week, allowing you to grab and go throughout the week and still eat healthy!

Fruit Salad

Fruit does not have to be boring! Try serving a fruit salad in your child's (or your own) lunch to see how exciting fruit can be.

- Kid Friendly Fruit Salad
- 2 red apples (your personal preference is fine)
- 1 sliced banana
- 1 green apple
- 2 pears
- Handful of red or green grapes
- Handful of slivered almonds
- 1 cup Greek yogurt, plain
- 2 teaspoons of cinnamon
- 3 teaspoons apple cider

Wash all of the fruits. Core and peel the apples and pears. Slice all fruit into bite size chunks. Place all fruit into a bowl. In a separate bowl combine yogurt, apple cider and cinnamon and pour over the fruit. Sprinkle with almonds and chill.

Beans and Rice

Beans and rice are a wonderful way to incorporate filling clean eating into your diet. Did you know that they make a delicious lunchtime salad? For kids that might balk at salads, you can also serve this recipe wrapped in a whole grain tortilla with clean eating guacamole or salsa.

- Delicious Bean and Rice Salad
- 2 cups cooked brown rice (cooled)
- ½ cups cooked black beans
- ¼ cup olive oil
- 2 fresh limes (or enough to make ¼ cup lime juice)
- 1 fresh tomato chopped
- 1 teaspoon garlic powder
- 1 teaspoon onion powder
- Fresh cilantro chopped (to taste)
- Pinch of salt and pepper (to taste)

Combine the rice, beans, chopped tomato and chopped cilantro in a bowl. In a separate bowl, combine the olive oil and lime juice, whisking until combined. Toss the bean/rice mixture with the dressing mixture and top with garlic powder, onion powder, salt and pepper.

**You can also add cooked chicken breast to this recipe, which is especially good if serving it in tortillas. Simply add the cooked chicken with the rice and beans and complete the recipe the same way.

Homemade Salsa

Stop purchasing store bought salsa that contains unnecessary preservatives! At the beginning of the week, make your own to serve on salads, tortillas and even whole grain chips.

- 4 medium sized tomatoes (organic if possible)
- 3 garlic cloves, minced
- 1 jalapeno pepper (or more if you prefer your salsa spicy)
- Chopped cilantro (to taste)
- 1 lime (juiced)
- Salt and pepper to taste

Chop the tomatoes and jalapenos as finely as possible. Mince the garlic and chop the cilantro as finely as possible too. Combine all ingredients and top with lime juice. Sprinkle with salt and pepper to taste. Chill for 2 hours before serving.

Not your Ordinary Chicken Salad

- 2 limes juiced
- 3 tablespoons olive oil
- 2 cloves garlic - crushed

- 1 teaspoon chili powder
- 2 cups chicken breasts, cooked
- 1 each red, green and yellow bell peppers, cut into thin strips
- 2 jalapeno peppers -- stemmed, seeded,
- 1 avocado, seeded, peeled and sliced

Salt and pepper to taste

Blend lime juice, oil, garlic, chili powder, salt and pepper in large bowl. Add chicken, sliced bell peppers and jalapenos. Add avocado chunks; toss lightly, and chill for 2 to 3 hours.

Green Salad with Chick Peas

It is amazing what the addition of nutrition packed chickpeas can do to an ordinary salad! Make this salad ahead of time and enjoy it at lunch.

- 1 head of lettuce of your choice, torn
- Organic cherry tomatoes, chopped
- 1 cup chickpeas, drained and rinsed
- ½ sliced red onion

Combine all ingredients and top with Balsamic Dressing (recipe below).

Balsamic Dressing

- 1/8 cup grapeseed or safflower oil (avoid olive oil for this recipe)
- 1/2 cup Balsamic vinegar
- 1 3/4 teaspoons Dijon mustard (read ingredients to make sure there's no added sugar)
- 1 teaspoon dried basil
- 2 teaspoons fresh parsley -- chopped
- 1 teaspoon dried oregano
- 1 teaspoon garlic powder

Combine the ingredients, mixing well. Add the vinegar slowly to allow you to adjust for personal taste. In a proper, air tight container, this could last for a few weeks.

For those days that you do not want to create a salad or you do not have the ingredients to make delicious bean and rice wraps – get creative! Kids love things that are served in shapes or even on a stick! Make it fun, with the following tips:

- Grapes and melon balls on a stick

- Cherry tomatoes and fresh mozzarella balls on a stick

- Cut whole grain bread with a cookie cutter and spread with natural peanut butter or nut butter

- Serve the colors of the rainbow in one container – strawberries, mandarin oranges, pineapple, green grapes, blueberries and plums or substitute any other clean eating foods to make the colors

- Hardboiled eggs make a great lunch

- Chickpeas roasted in the oven with a sprinkling of salt is a delicious crunchy side for lunch

- Homemade applesauce (recipe to follow)

- Make a sandwich out of apple slices, peanut butter and granola

- Send the fixings for a salad, including lettuce, tomatoes, sliced carrots, almonds, chickpeas, cucumbers and homemade dressing and let them fix it themselves

All of these ideas work for kids and adults and can be altered to meet your own dietary restrictions and/or preferences. The key is to have fun!

Make Your Own Applesauce

While it can be tempting to purchase one of the many varieties of applesauce at the grocery store, a quick look at the label will tell you that it probably contains high fructose corn syrup or another additive that is unnecessary. Making your own applesauce is not as daunting as it sounds and it tastes delicious.

Homemade Applesauce

- 3 pounds of sweet apples (your preference)
- Enough water to cover the apples when cooking
- Dash of fresh lemon juice
- Cinnamon, to taste

Wash, core and peel your apples, then chop them into bite size chunks. Place them in a large pot and cover with water. Do not completely submerge all of the apples, just add enough water to reach almost to the top. Add lemon juice and cinnamon to taste and bring to a boil. Once boiling, reduce the heat to medium and let the apples cook until they are completely soft and can be mashed. Once cooked, you can mash it by hand or place in the blender. Once it is completely smooth, store the applesauce in an air tight container in the refrigerator.

Dinner

Clean eating dinners, even for the busiest family, can be easily to accomplish. There are not a lot of ingredients and the cooking methods are rather simple. Following are a few simple recipes for you to use as a basis to get your ideas flowing for clean eating dinners. Sometimes it helps families to come up with themes to make dinner preparation easier. Below is a sample theme format that you can adapt for your own uses:

Meatless Monday – Introduce a meatless option for your family, you might be surprised how much everyone enjoys these meals as much as those filled with meat

Taco Tuesday – Experiment with different ways to serve tacos including with ground turkey and chicken

Wacky Wednesday – Make Wednesday the day that you all try something completely new

Time for Leftovers Thursday – Don't be wasteful, save time and eat the leftovers from the week

Fajita Friday – Fajitas are as versatile as tacos and can be served many different ways

Sandwich Saturday – Take a break on Saturdays and serve wholesome sandwiches

Sunday is a Funday – Sunday is the day for family and gatherings, make the meal that your family loves the most.

Ideas for Meatless Monday

For most people, thinking of ways to serve a satisfying dinner without meat can be difficult, but it is not impossible. Try to think outside of the box using ingredients such as whole grain pasta, rice, beans, spinach, whole grain pizza crust, stir fry, soup or serve breakfast for dinner! Once you get used to serving meals without meat – Meatless Mondays can become fun.

Here are a few examples of what you can serve:

- Whole grain pasta and spinach drizzled with olive oil and parmesan cheese
- Bean and rice burritos made with whole grain tortillas
- Vegetable stir fry made with brown rice
- Vegetable soup
- Whole Grain Pasta with Spinach
- 1 pound whole grain pasta
- 1 bunch fresh spinach, torn
- 3 garlic cloves, minced
- ½ cup olive oil
- ½ cup parmesan cheese

Cook the pasta as the directions state. In another pan, heat the olive oil and sauté the garlic until slightly brown. Once the pasta is cooked, drain it and place the spinach leaves on top of the pasta. Dump the pasta and spinach back into the pan, to allow the spinach leaves to heat up. Once back in the pan, toss the olive oil and garlic mixture over the top, mixing well. Top with parmesan cheese and serve.

Bean and Rice Tortillas

Using the recipe above for Bean and Rice Salad, you can make Bean and Rice Tortillas. Simply add whole grain tortillas, homemade salsa and homemade guacamole and you have a delicious Mexican feast that is meatless and clean eating!

Vegetable Stir Fry

The wonderful thing about stir fry, whether you are making it for Meatless Monday and including only veggies or you are making it later in the week with a protein, is the versatility of the dish. You can change it virtually every time that you make it, giving your family a new opportunity to try different things every week. For Meatless Monday, you can stick with a few basic vegetables and then add a new one each week to give everyone the chance to experiment a little bit.

- Basic Veggie Stir Fry
- Red, green and yellow bell peppers
- Bean sprouts
- Broccoli
- Mushrooms
- 2 garlic cloves, minced
- ½ white onion, diced
- Brown rice or quinoa
- 2 tablespoon coconut oil

Heat the coconut oil in a large pan. Once hot, add the minced garlic and onion and cook until slightly brown. Lower the heat slightly and add the vegetables that you have chosen, including the above and any additions that you are using. Sauté the vegetables until they are al dente. In the meantime, cook the brown rice or quinoa as directed. Serve the vegetables over the rice or quinoa and enjoy!

**If you or your kids prefer soy sauce over your stir fry, use minimal amounts of reduced sodium soy sauce.

Make Taco Tuesday Fun

Taco Tuesday can be a really fun way to celebrate Tuesday in your house. There are endless ways to serve tacos to ensure that no one gets bored; in fact many households use Taco Tuesday as a way to incorporate everyone in the kitchen at least one day a week.

There are various proteins that you can use for tacos including: lean chicken breast, lean ground meat, lean ground turkey and veggies. So start your Taco night by choosing the protein of the week. They can all be prepared in almost the same way, with the exception of the veggie tacos. For chicken, ground beef and ground turkey use the following method:

Pour a small amount of olive oil in a large pan. Heat the olive oil for a minute or two, until hot and add your protein. If you are using chicken breasts, make sure to slice them into bite sizes pieces before adding to the pan. Cook the meat all the way through and then add your seasonings and a couple of tablespoons of water. It is easiest if you make a large batch of taco seasoning ahead of time because then you can just sprinkle a liberal amount right on your protein. If you do not make it in bulk, then you can sprinkle each spice in the following recipe on individually.

Homemade Taco Seasoning

You can alter this recipe to meet your own preferences, but this is a good starter recipe to use until you figure out what your family likes. Making your own taco seasoning is not only economical, but it is also much healthier because you know exactly what is going into the seasoning and you know there are no additives or harmful chemicals.

Taco Seasoning

- 3 teaspoons chili powder
- 1 ¼ teaspoon cumin
- 1 teaspoon paprika
- 1 teaspoon salt
- ½ teaspoon oregano
- ¾ teaspoon garlic powder
- ¼ teaspoon onion powder
- ¼ - ½ red pepper flakes

Mix all of the ingredients together and store in an airtight container. You can use as much or as little of the spice that you want on your meat, the average amount is 2 to 3 tablespoons per pound of meat.

Once you have your meat cooked, there are many ways to serve your tacos:

- Standard tacos with whole grain taco shells – Serve with chopped tomatoes, chopped avocado, shredded lettuce and homemade salsa
- Taco salad – Serve your protein over a bed of a variety of lettuce, include whole grain tortilla strips, homemade salsa, avocado slices, black beans, sliced red onions and chopped tomatoes
- "Untacos" – Rather than using taco shells, use large pieces of lettuce as a wrap for all of the taco fixings

•Taco casserole – Use the same ingredients as above, but layer them in a casserole

Chicken Kabobs

Another great way to try new veggies is to serve them on a stick! Make chicken kabobs often, simply change out the veggies that you use. This will give everyone a chance to try a new veggie in an enticing way.

Marinade

Start by slicing and marinating your chicken in this delicious recipe:

- 2 tablespoons olive oil
- 1 teaspoon paprika
- 1 ½ teaspoon garlic powder
- ½ teaspoon savory
- ½ teaspoon onion powder
- ½ teaspoon dried basil

Place all ingredients in a Ziploc bag and swish around until thoroughly covered. Place your chicken in the refrigerator for at least 2 hours to allow the flavors to meld.

Kabobs

Once the chicken is marinated, choose your veggies and slice them into 2-inch cubes. A few great choices include:

- Broccoli
- Onions
- Mushrooms
- Zucchini
- Eggplant
- Any color bell pepper
- Fennel
- Carrots
- Tomatoes
- Asparagus

You can try almost any veggie – let your kids choose some to try! Grill your kabobs and enjoy! If you do not want to grill them, they can also be placed in a 350 degree oven on a parchment lined pan. Make sure to flip them halfway through cooking. It usually takes about 10 minutes per side for the meat to cook through.

Homemade Bread Crumbs

Clean eating does not mean that you have to give up some of your favorite recipes, such as chicken parmesan, chicken nuggets or breaded fish, it just means that you need to find ways to adapt. One of the best ways is to make your own breadcrumbs. It is not as hard as it sounds and can be done in large batches. The amount of chemicals and preservatives that you will be avoiding are well worth the extra work!

Clean Eating Whole Grain Bread Crumbs

Whole grain bread (use the ends of bread that you normally throw out or bread that is past its prime)

- Cookie Sheet
- Food Processor or Blender
- Optional Ingredients
- Garlic Powder
- Oregano
- Parmesan Cheese

Lay the bread out on a cookie sheet and cook in a 250 degree oven until it dries out. This usually takes between 20 and 30 minutes. Keep an eye on your bread and adjust the time accordingly. Let them cool and then throw them in the blender or food processor to create your bread crumbs. This provides nutritious (preservative free) plain bread crumbs. You can modify them with the above spices in any quantity or any other spices that your family prefers. Store the crumbs in an airtight container. They keep for up to 6 months in the freezer.

Chicken Fajitas

Fajitas are a wonderful way to sneak in veggies and still have a fun dinner. Kids love the vibrant colors of the various peppers and parents love the delicious taste of this Mexican treat. If you make your own seasoning and purchase whole grain or corn tortillas, it can be an easy clean eating meal!

Delicious Chicken Fajitas

- 4 boneless, skinless chicken breasts sliced
- Bell peppers in a variety of colors, sliced
- 2 onions, sliced
- 2 teaspoons lime juice
- 1 ½ teaspoons olive oil
- 2 teaspoons cumin
- 2 teaspoons chili powder
- 1 teaspoon garlic powder
- Corn or whole grain tortillas (no sugar added)

Heat the olive oil in a large pan and add the chicken, half of the lime juice and half of each of the spices. Cook 4 minutes on each side or until cooked through. Remove the chicken and replace with the onions and peppers. Sprinkle with the remaining spices and lime juice and cook until tender. Place the chicken back with the vegetables and heat through. Serve with homemade salsa and guacamole.

Roasted Vegetables

Another great way to get kids to eat vegetables (and like them) is to roast them. This method takes very few ingredients and yet brings out a natural sweetness in the vegetables that make kids eat them, no matter how much they did not like them before. A few great ones to try are broccoli, cauliflower and asparagus – but you can try almost any vegetable this way!

Roasted Veggies

- 1 head broccoli, cauliflower or bunch of asparagus
- 2 tablespoons of olive oil
- 3 tablespoons parmesan cheese

Wash and dry the vegetable. Lay it out in an even layer on a cookie sheet. Sprinkle with olive oil and parmesan cheese. Place in a 400 degree oven for 20 minutes or until crispy. Enjoy!

Chapter 10 – You Did It!

As you can hopefully see, clean eating does not have to be too difficult and it can even be fun! Even the busiest families can find a way to incorporate one or more clean eating techniques into their daily routine in order to encourage optimal health in all of your family members. Remember to take it one step at a time and truly enjoy the journey.

Clean eating is meant to be a way to bring your eating habits back to the basics and back to a time that you were able to enjoy the true taste of foods, the way that they were meant to be enjoyed.

When you stop and think about the advertisements and line of thinking that food manufacturers have made us all believe, you will see how easy it was to get caught up in eating processed foods.

Now that you know the truth about the food that you have been eating, it will be easier to take them out of your life. If you have young kids, make sure to include them in all of the decisions, shopping and cooking. Let them truly learn how important good nutrition is and show them just how they can achieve that good nutrition by making the right food choices.

Hopefully this book has helped you to want to make some changes in your family's eating habits, whether it is one change or a lot of changes. Even baby steps are better than continuing the bad eating habits that are currently used by any family. Take the time to recognize the small steps that you take and enjoy the journey of clean eating. Chances are that once you start the journey, you will love how you feel and love the taste of the food, making you want to incorporate even more changes to your diet down the road.

References

Levy, J., LM Segal, K. Thomas, R. St. Laurent, A. Lang, and J. Rayburn. "F as in Fat: How Obesity Threatens America's Future 2013." RWJF. N.p., n.d. Web. 14 May 2014.

"University News Service." Study: No-fat, Low-fat Dressings Don't Get Most Nutrients out of Salads. N.p., n.d. Web. 14 May 2014.

32613448R00057

Printed in Great Britain
by Amazon